UTERINE FIBROIDS COOKBOOK FOR NEWLY DIAGNOSED

Discover Nutritional Solutions, Proven Strategies, Meal Plans, Medical Insights, And Lifestyle Tips To For Managing Uterine Fibroids Naturally

DR. ERIC TRISTAN

CONTENTS

DISCLAIMER

The information provided in this book, is intended for informational purposes only. The content is not intended to be a substitute for professional medical advice, diagnosis, or treatment. Always seek the advice of your physician or other qualified health provider with any questions you may have regarding a medical condition. Never disregard professional medical advice or delay in seeking it because of something you have read in this book.

The author of this book has made reasonable efforts to ensure that the information provided is accurate and up-to-date at the time of publication. However, the author makes no representations or warranties of any kind, express or implied, about the completeness, accuracy, reliability, suitability, or availability of the information contained within these pages.

Any reliance you place on the information provided in this book is strictly at your own risk. The author shall not be liable for any loss, injury, or damage arising from the use of this book or the information contained herein.

The mention or reference to any individuals, products, websites, organizations, or other names within this book does not imply endorsement by the author. The inclusion of such references is solely for informational purposes and does not constitute an endorsement or recommendation.

Furthermore, the author disclaims any association or affiliation with any individuals, products, websites, organizations, or other names mentioned in this book.

It is important to consult with a qualified healthcare professional before making any dietary or lifestyle changes, especially if you have a medical condition. Each individual's health situation is unique, and what works for one person may not work for another.

Again, the information provided in this book is not intended to diagnose, treat, cure, or prevent any disease or health condition. Always seek the advice of a physician or other qualified health provider regarding any medical questions or concerns you may have.

Thank you for your understanding and for taking the necessary precautions when considering the information presented in this book.

ABOUT THIS BOOK

This "Uterine Fibroids Cookbook" is an exceptional resource that assists individuals in understanding the intricacies of uterine fibroids by offering a thorough examination of dietary selections and lifestyle modifications that may have a beneficial effect on uterine health. This book begins with a scholarly introduction that establishes the context for an examination of the foundational aspects of uterine fibroids and the complex correlation between diet and these conditions. Through an exploration of the intricate correlation between diet and uterine fibroids, this book emphasizes the criticality of exercising knowledge when selecting foods to consume.

The table of contents exhibits a judicious arrangement, commencing with a fundamental comprehension of uterine fibroids and progressively advancing to pragmatic suggestions. This book provides practical and concise advice in chapters such as "Foods to Include for Uterine Health" and "Foods to Avoid for Uterine Health," enabling readers to make well-informed decisions regarding their daily dietary selections. By incorporating a wide variety of nourishing recipes suitable for breakfast, lunch, dinner, snacking, and desserts, this program guarantees a varied and pleasurable method of promoting uterine health via gastronomic selections. This not only considers the dietary component but also accommodates the diverse inclinations and ways of life of the audience.

The inclusion of strategies for meal planning and preparation serves to augment the pragmatic value of this book, enabling the effortless assimilation of practices that are beneficial for the uterus into routine activities. Through the inclusion of botanicals, supplements, and lifestyle modifications, this book offers a comprehensive perspective on uterine health. The incorporation of mindful dining practices cultivates a more profound correlation between dietary choices and holistic health.

The inclusion of sample meal plans and a dedicated section providing answers to frequently asked questions enhances the practicality of the content, offering readers practical guidance and addressing prevalent concerns.

The "Uterine Fibroids Cookbook" serves as an indispensable resource for individuals who desire to adopt a proactive and knowledgeable strategy in overseeing uterine health via dietary adjustments and changes to their way of life. The exhaustive nature of the resource, supported by a lucid and structured table of contents, establishes it as an essential instrument in the pursuit of uterine health.

CHAPTER ONE

A Brief Overview Of The Uterine Fibroids Cookbook

Uterine fibroids are benign uterine growths that frequently manifest during the period of childbearing. Although these growths are typically noncancerous, they have the potential to induce discomfort and may hurt fertility. Managing uterine fibroids requires a holistic approach, and the significance of diet is an element that is frequently disregarded. To tackle this issue, The Uterine Fibroids Cookbook presents a dietary manual that is customized to suit the dietary needs of individuals afflicted with uterine fibroids.

Comprehension Of Uterine Fibroids

Before exploring the fundamentals of the cookbook, it is critical to acquire knowledge about uterine fibroids. These protuberances, alternatively referred to as leiomyomas or myomas, originate from the myomas of the uterus. In addition to pressure on the bladder or rectum, they may cause excessive menstrual bleeding, pelvic discomfort, and variation in size and quantity.

Although the precise etiology of uterine fibroids is unknown, their development may be influenced by hormonal factors, genetic predisposition, and environmental elements. A comprehensive comprehension of the determinants that impact fibroid proliferation is imperative for the successful management thereof.

A multifaceted strategy is required to manage uterine fibroids, including dietary modifications, lifestyle adjustments, and medical interventions. The Uterine Fibroids Cookbook places particular emphasis on the latter, acknowledging the potential importance of nutrition in the management of fibroid symptoms and its influence on overall health.

Dietary Influence On Uterine Fibroids

Regarding the management of uterine fibroids, the impact of diet on hormonal equilibrium and inflammation levels is substantial. While some foods may exacerbate fibroid symptoms by contributing to hormonal imbalances, others may have the potential to alleviate such symptoms. A diet abundant in nutrients that promote hormonal homeostasis and reduce inflammation is emphasized in the cookbook.

Maintaining a healthy weight is a critical component, given that obesity is correlated with an elevated likelihood of developing fibroid and experiencing a worsening of symptoms. A well-balanced diet consisting of an assortment of fruits, vegetables, whole cereals, and lean proteins is recommended in the cookbook. These dietary items are rich in vital vitamins and minerals, which contribute to overall well-being and potentially aid in the regulation of hormones.

Specific dietary constituents may exert a direct influence on estrogen levels, a hormone that is known to affect the proliferation of fibroid tissue. Phytoestrogens, which are present in plant-based foods including soy products, potentially possess anti-estrogenic and estrogen-like properties, thereby aiding in the regulation of hormonal activity. The compendium presents recipes that integrate these healthful foods, thereby offering a pragmatic approach to integrating them into routine dietary regimens.

The cookbook not only discusses hormone management but also inflammation, which is a contributing factor to a range of health conditions, including fibroids. Berry pulp, verdant greens, and oily fish that are abundant in omega-3 fatty acids are recommended as anti-inflammatory foods. Potential benefits of consuming these foods include inflammation reduction and symptomatic relief from uterine fibroids.

Included Foods For Uterine Health

The Uterine Fibroids Cookbook presents an exhaustive enumeration of dietary components that individuals afflicted with uterine fibroids ought to incorporate into their regimen to effectively manage symptoms and promote uterine health.

1. Fruits and vegetables are the cornerstone of a diet that is beneficial for individuals with fibroid syndrome due to their abundance of vitamins, minerals, and antioxidants. A variety of nutrients present in leafy greens, cruciferous vegetables, and vibrant fruits promote overall health and potentially aid in hormonal regulation.

2. Whole grains, including quinoa, brown rice, and oatmeal, are nutritionally dense and rich in vital nutrients and fiber. In addition to being essential for digestive health, fiber may also aid in weight management, which is a critical component of fibroid treatment.

3. The consumption of lean proteins, including those found in poultry, fish, legumes, and tofu, is crucial for maintaining optimal muscle health and overall wellness. Additionally, protein aids in the maintenance of hormonal equilibrium.

4. The cookbook prioritizes foods that are abundant in omega-3 fatty acids, including salmon, walnuts,

and flaxseeds. Anti-inflammatory in nature, these lipids may assist in reducing the inflammation that is linked to fibroids.

5. The compendium comprises recipes that highlight foods abundant in phytoestrogens, such as sesame seeds, flaxseeds, and soy products. These nutrients potentially aid in the regulation of estrogen levels and promote hormonal equilibrium.

6. Specific herbs and seasonings that are renowned for their anti-inflammatory attributes are integrated into the recipes found in the cookbook. For instance, turmeric, ginger, and garlic may offer supplementary assistance in the management of inflammation.

In summary, the Uterine Fibroids Cookbook functions as an invaluable asset for individuals who are confronted with the complexities associated with uterine fibroids. By gaining a comprehension of the condition, acknowledging the influence of diet on fibroid symptoms, and integrating particular foods into their daily diets, individuals can adopt a proactive stance in the management of uterine fibroids and the enhancement of uterine health as a whole. By integrating nutrition with other facets of fibroid management, this comprehensive strategy enables people to maximize their health and improve their overall quality of life.

Avoided Foods For Uterine Health

Uterine fibroids, which frequently manifest during the reproductive years and are benign growths in the uterus, are amenable to a combination of medical interventions and modifications to one's lifestyle, such as dietary modifications. The objective of The Uterine Fibroids Cookbook is to assist women who are managing this condition by offering recommendations on which foods should be excluded to promote optimal uterine health.

Highly processed foods frequently comprise artificial ingredients, preservatives, and additives that have the potential to disturb the equilibrium of hormones. These substances have the potential to promote the development and proliferation of uterine fibroids. The cookbook advocates for the avoidance of packaged munchies, high-trans-fat fast food, and sugary desserts.

Dairy Products and Red Meat: Hormones and pesticides found in high-fat dairy products and red meat have the potential to disrupt the body's hormonal regulation. It is recommended in the cookbook to restrict the intake of full-fat dairy products and instead choose lean sources of protein, such as poultry or plant-based substitutes.

Overindulgence in refined carbohydrates and sweets has the potential to induce inflammation and worsen hormonal imbalances that are commonly linked to uterine fibroids. To promote optimal uterine health, the cookbook advises reducing the consumption of desserts, chocolates, and sugary beverages to a minimum.

Caffeine and alcohol have the potential to influence hormone levels and may also promote inflammation. It is recommended in the cookbook that women who have uterine fibroids restrict their consumption of caffeinated beverages, such as coffee, and alcohol to foster a more balanced hormonal environment.

Elevated Sodium Content: Dietary sources abundant in sodium may contribute to water retention and edema, which may exacerbate the symptoms linked to uterine fibroids. A reduction in the consumption of processed and salty foods is recommended in the cookbook as a means to mitigate these concerns and promote holistic uterine health.

CHAPTER TWO

Recipes And Nutrients For Uterine Fibroids

To promote uterine health, the Uterine Fibroids Cookbook emphasizes the incorporation of nutrient-dense ingredients into recipes, as opposed to foods to avoid.

By integrating these components into one's dietary regimen, one can initiate beneficial measures to regulate uterine fibroids and promote holistic health.

For uterine health recipes, verdant greens such as kale, spinach, and collard greens are excellent inclusions because they are rich in vitamins and minerals. The high fiber content of these vegetables can aid in the regulation of hormonal equilibrium and the reduction of inflammation.

Antioxidants, which are abundant in colorful fruits such as berries and citrus fruits, are of critical importance in the fight against oxidative stress and inflammation.

This cookbook promotes the incorporation of an assortment of fruits to guarantee a varied supply of nutrients that are beneficial for uterine health.

Selecting whole grains rather than refined grains facilitates the maintenance of consistent energy levels and aids in the regulation of insulin. Whole cereals such as quinoa, brown rice, and oats are featured in the cookbook and can be incorporated into recipes for breakfast, lunch, and supper.

Incorporating lean protein sources into one's diet, such as poultry, fish, tofu, and legumes, promotes muscle health and aids in weight maintenance. The cookbook features recipes that effectively highlight these proteins in scrumptious and nourishing amalgamations.

Health Benefits of Healthy Fats: Essential fatty acids, which are abundant in almonds, avocados, and olive oil, are vital for maintaining hormonal equilibrium.

The Uterine Fibroids Cookbook comprises recipes that integrate these beneficial lipids to promote uterine health as a whole.

Early Morning Delights

Breakfast that is both nutritious and well-balanced establishes an ideal beginning to the day, furnishing individuals with the necessary energy and nutrients to uphold their overall health, with particular emphasis on those who are tasked with managing uterine fibroids. Breakfast recipes in The Uterine Fibroids Cookbook are expertly crafted to promote uterine health.

Smoothie bowls are an appetizing and practical breakfast alternative due to their inclusion of protein sources such as Greek yogurt or plant-based protein powder, nutrient-dense fruits, and verdant vegetables. The cookbook offers innovative amalgamations that accommodate diverse gustatory inclinations.

Variations on Oatmeal: Oats made with whole grains are an adaptable foundation for a nourishing breakfast. Oatmeal recipes incorporating garnishes like fresh berries, almonds, and seeds are included in the cookbook to aid in nutrient absorption and morning satiety.

Egg-Based Dishes: Eggs possess exceptional protein content and can be seamlessly integrated into a multitude of breakfast preparations. The cookbook comprises delectable and protein-rich omelet, frittata, and egg muffin recipes, providing a gratifying and nutritious beginning to the day.

Yogurt parfaits are an appetizing and nourishing breakfast option, composed of granola, almonds, and vibrant fruits spread over Greek yogurt. Combinations recommended in the Uterine Fibroids Cookbook not only promote uterine health but also accommodate personal taste preferences.

Lunch To Promote Uterine Health

Lunch serves as a pivotal occasion to replenish vitality and establish a solid foundation for the remainder of the day.

The lunch recipes in The Uterine Fibroids Cookbook emphasize the use of nutrient-dense components to promote uterine health.

Salads containing Protein: An all-around salad comprising vibrant vegetables, verdant greens, lean protein, and a wholesome vinaigrette can serve as a gratifying and healthful repast for two. A wide array of salad recipes is featured in the cookbook to infuse lunchtime with variety and flavor.

Whole grain wraps provide a portable and well-balanced lunch alternative by incorporating a variety of vegetables, lean proteins, and whole grains. The cookbook comprises a selection of recipes that highlight diverse flavor characteristics, thereby guaranteeing an array of options to accommodate personal inclinations.

Lunch Recipes Loaded with Plant-Based and Vegetarian Proteins, Including Tofu, Lentils, and Beans, the Uterine Fibroids Cookbook provides suggestions for individuals following a plant-based or vegetarian diet. These alternatives offer vital nutrients while advocating for a dietary regimen that emphasizes uterine health.

Soup and Stew Varieties: Soups and stews that are rich in nutrients can serve as nourishing and comforting options for lunch. The cookbook features a selection of recipes that incorporate lean proteins, whole cereals, and an assortment of vegetables to promote uterine health.

Recipes For Dinners That Promote Uterine Health

In the late hours of the day, dinner presents an occasion to savor a gratifying and nourishing supper that promotes the well-being of the uterus. The Uterine Fibroids Cookbook is an anthology of dinner recipes that emphasize the use of essential ingredients that promote holistic health.

Salmon, which is fatty and abundant in omega-3 fatty acids, can be an excellent complement to supper preparations when grilled or baked. The cookbook offers inventive methods for preparing fish that has been grilled or roasted, guaranteeing a delectable and nutritionally dense meal.

Frying colorful vegetables in stir-fries that include lean protein sources and flavorful seasonings can produce a scrumptious and expeditious supper. The cookbook features stir-fry recipes that highlight an assortment of vegetables that are known to promote uterine health.

Quinoa and Vegetable dishes: Quinoa, an adaptable whole grain, functions as the foundation for fortifying dishes brimming with vibrant vegetables, lean sources of protein, and nutritious fats. The cookbook provides customizable recipes that accommodate specific personal preferences and dietary restrictions.

Pasta substitutes derived from whole grains or legumes offer a scrumptious and nutrient-dense basis for an assortment of dinner recipes. Pasta dishes in The Uterine Fibroids Cookbook integrate colorful vegetables and lean proteins to compose a nutritionally balanced meal.

To summarize, the Uterine Fibroids Cookbook is an invaluable resource for women who are interested in utilizing dietary modifications to manage uterine fibroids. By integrating foods that are abundant in essential nutrients and avoiding those that have the potential to worsen symptoms, individuals can adopt a proactive stance in safeguarding the health of their uterus.

By prioritizing a wide range of delectable breakfast, lunch, and dinner recipes, the cookbook guarantees a holistic strategy for attaining holistic well-being while dealing with uterine fibroids.

CHAPTER THREE

Alternative Snacks For Uterine Fibroids

Uterine fibroids are benign protuberances located in the uterus that may induce pain and a range of other symptoms. Although a definitive dietary regimen to cure or prevent fibroids does not exist, specific foods may aid in symptom management and promote uterine health as a whole. Individuals with uterine fibroids must consume refreshments that are rich in nutrients and promote a healthy lifestyle.

1. The inclusion of almonds and seeds in one's refreshment regimen may have advantageous effects on uterine health. Omega-3 fatty acids, which are abundant in flaxseeds, walnuts, and almonds, possess anti-inflammatory properties. Moreover, they furnish vital nutrients such as zinc and magnesium, thereby making a significant contribution to holistic health.

2. Greek Yogurt with Berries: Protein and calcium, both of which are essential for bone health, are abundant in Greek yogurt. Berry additions that are abundant in antioxidants, such as strawberries and blueberries, not only improve flavor but also supply the immune system with vitamins and minerals.

3. Combining hummus with vibrant vegetable spears, including carrots, cucumber, and bell peppers, for a snack, presents a gratifying and healthful alternative. The fiber present in vegetables facilitates digestion, whereas hummus provides protein and healthful lipids.

4. Chia seed pudding is an excellent source of omega-3 fatty acids and fiber. When combined with almond milk and allowed to develop, the result is a texture resembling pudding. In addition to being delectable, this refreshment is rich in nutrients that are advantageous to uterine health.

5. Avocado toast made with whole-grain bread contains potassium and monounsaturated lipids.

Apply it onto whole grain bread to increase fiber intake. Whole grains are known to promote cardiovascular health and potentially offer relief from the symptoms associated with fibroid.

6. Air-popped popcorn seasoned with turmeric has the potential to serve as a delectable and anti-inflammatory refreshment option. Curcumin, which is present in turmeric, has been recognized for its capacity to mitigate inflammation and enhance general well-being.

7. Incorporating a variety of fruits into a revitalizing salad containing mint can serve as both a delicious and nutritious refreshment. Additionally to imparting a surge of flavor, mint may also aid digestion.

8. Smoothie Bowls: Construct a nourishing smoothie bowl by combining fruits, vegetables, and a protein source, such as plant-based protein powder or Greek yogurt. This refreshment alternative fosters ingenuity while guaranteeing an equilibrium of vital nutrients.

9. Young soybeans, or edamame, are an excellent source of plant-based protein. Furthermore, their fiber and antioxidant content contributes to their healthiness as a whole refreshment.

10.Nuts and Dark Chocolate: Dark chocolate, when consumed in moderation, can be an enjoyable indulgence. Nuts should be added for added texture and nutritional value. The antioxidant content of dark chocolate suggests that it might have mood-boosting properties.

Although these sustenance options are regarded as uterine-friendly, it is still imperative to uphold a well-rounded diet comprising an assortment of foods. Beyond that, it is advisable to seek personalized guidance from a healthcare professional.

Desserts Suitable For The Uterine System

It is of the utmost importance to incorporate a diet that promotes overall health when managing uterine fibroids. Although a definitive "uterine fibroids cookbook" does not exist, integrating desserts that adhere to a uterine-friendly diet can provide both gratification and promote overall health. The following confection suggestions feature nutrient-dense components that may aid in the management of fibroid symptoms:

1. Berry and Yogurt Parfait: A delectable and nourishing dessert is produced by alternating layers of Greek yogurt and assorted fruit. Antioxidants are abundant in berries, whereas probiotics and protein found in Greek yogurt promote digestive health.

2. Baked Apples with Cinnamon: A warm and comforting delicacy, baked apples dusted with cinnamon. The anti-inflammatory properties of cinnamon and the fiber content of apples may assist in the management of uterine fibroid symptoms.

3. Fresh Fruit with Chia Seed Pudding Chia seed pudding is a versatile dessert base. Incorporate fresh fruits such as kiwis, mangoes, or berries on top to

impart additional nutrients, minerals, and a naturally occurring flavor.

4. Produce an opulent and velvety chocolate mousse by putting to use mature avocados. By the antioxidants in cocoa powder and the healthful fats in avocados, this confection is both decadent and nutrient-dense.

5. Oatmeal Banana Cookies: For a straightforward and nutritious cookie recipe, blend pureed bananas with oatmeal. With the fiber and potassium provided by bananas and bananas, respectively, these pastries are a guilt-free sweet delight.

6. Coconut Date Balls: Prepare a nutritious snack by combining dates, coconut, and almonds in a blender. Dates impart an inherent sweetness, whereas pistachios and coconut provide nutritious lipids and vital nutrients, respectively.

7. Frozen Yogurt Bark: Spread a mixture of Greek yogurt and your preferred fruits onto a baking sheet and place in the freezer. Once it has hardened, sever

it into segments to create a fruity and refreshing frozen delight.

8. Quinoa Pudding: Bring quinoa and almond milk to a simmer before adding a dash of honey or maple syrup for sweetness. With the addition of almond milk and quinoa, which are both complete proteins, a nourishing confection is produced.

9. To prepare a revitalizing sorbet, combine pomegranate seeds with a small amount of honey and place the mixture in the freezer. Antioxidants abound in pomegranates, which potentially impart anti-inflammatory properties.

10. To enhance the nutritional value of banana bread, substitute hazelnuts for their crunchiness and omega-3 fatty acid content. By substituting whole wheat flour and reducing added sugars, this confection could be made more welcoming to the uterus.

Exercise moderation when consuming desserts and maintain a mindful approach to one's overall dietary decisions. Furthermore, seeking advice from a healthcare professional can offer tailored recommendations that are specific to an individual's health requirements.

CHAPTER FOUR

Fluids Beneficial To Uterine Health

Sustaining uterine health necessitates conscientious decision-making about both dietary and beverage selection. Although no beverage can provide a definitive cure or preventative measure against uterine fibroids, consuming beverages that are abundant in specific nutrients may have a positive impact on overall health. Consider the following beverages regarding uterine health:

1. Herbal Teas: Herbal teas that contain potentially anti-inflammatory and soothing properties include chamomile, peppermint, and ginger. Particularly renowned for its tranquil properties, chamomile may assist in the management of tension.

2. Green Tea Green tea, specifically catechins, is an excellent source of antioxidants. Antioxidants potentially possess anti-inflammatory properties and consistent ingestion of green tea has been linked to a multitude of health advantages.

3. Latte Made with Turmeric: Curcumin, which is present in turmeric, has anti-inflammatory properties. A latte made with alternative milk, turmeric, and ginger has the potential to be both palatable and nutritionally beneficial.

4. Maintaining adequate hydration is vital for one's overall health. In addition to enhancing the flavor of water, adding a squeeze of lemon provides a measure of vitamin C, an essential nutrient for the immune system.

5. Pomegranate juice is an excellent source of antioxidants, specifically anthocyanins and polyphenols. Potentially possessing anti-inflammatory properties, these compounds may promote cardiovascular health in general.

6. Cranberry juice is recognized for its prospective health benefits to the urinary tract. Although further investigation is warranted, preliminary research indicates that cranberries might offer some protection against particular infections.

7. Smoothies Containing Leafy Greens: For a nutrient-dense beverage, incorporate leafy greens such as kale or spinach into a smoothie. Vitamins, minerals, and antioxidants found in leafy greens are beneficial to overall health.

8. Coconut water is an option that is both hydrating and abundant in electrolytes. Additionally, it is a revitalizing option due to its potassium content, which may aid in maintaining electrolyte balance.

9. Nitrates, which are abundant in beetroot juice, potentially offer cardiovascular advantages. Beetroot juice has the potential to be a nourishing and invigorating beverage that promotes general health.

10. An infusion of water infused with cucumber and mint leaves and segments produces a beverage that is both invigorating and rehydrating. Cucumbers offer hydration and are low in calories, whereas mint potentially possesses digestive advantages.

Individuals may react differently to beverages; therefore, moderation is essential. Furthermore, it is advisable to seek personalized guidance from a healthcare professional, particularly for individuals who are managing specific health conditions such as uterine fibroids.

Advice On Meal Preparation And Planning

Meal preparation and organization play a critical role in sustaining a healthy lifestyle, particularly for those coping with uterine fibroids. Although a definitive diet to cure or prevent fibroids does not exist, incorporating a balanced meal planning strategy can enhance general health and potentially aid in symptom management. The following are suggestions for meal preparation and planning in consideration of uterine health:

1. Make Whole Foods Your Top Priority: Provide your meals with nutrient-dense, whole foods. Diversify your dietary intake by including a selection of fruits, vegetables, whole cereals, lean proteins, and healthy lipids.

These dietary items are rich in vital nutrients that promote holistic well-being.

2. Incorporate Foods Rich in Fiber: Fiber is essential for healthy digestion. Consisting of a diverse array of foods abundant in fiber, such as fruits, vegetables, legumes, and whole grains, can aid in the maintenance of digestive health and promote regular bowel movements.

3. Select Lean Protein Sources: Lean protein sources, including poultry, fish, tofu, legumes, and seeds, should be prioritized. Protein is critical for the maintenance and repair of muscle tissue, and opting for lean protein sources can positively impact aerobic fitness.

4. Integrate Anti-Inflammatory Components: Incorporate ingredients renowned for their pro-inflammatory attributes, including olive oil, turmeric, ginger, and oily salmon abundant in omega-3 fatty acids. The inflammation associated with uterine fibroids may be alleviated by these.

5. It is advisable to restrict the consumption of manufactured foods and foods that are rich in added carbohydrates. These have the potential to exacerbate inflammation and have adverse effects on overall health.

6. Maintaining sufficient hydration is vital for one's overall health. Consume copious amounts of water daily and contemplate integrating hydrating foods into your diet, such as fruits and vegetables that are abundant in water.

7. Strive to organize well-balanced meals by incorporating a variety of nutrients—protein, healthy lipids, and carbohydrates—into your meal plan. This equilibrium contributes to the regulation of blood glucose levels and sustains energy.

8. Conducting Experiments with Herbs and Spices: Rather than relying excessively on salt, augment the flavor of your meals by utilizing herbs and spices. Herbs and seasonings such as rosemary, basil, and

thyme, in addition to cumin and cardamom, can impart complexity to your dishes.

9. It is important to exercise portion control to prevent excessive consumption. By attending to the signals of appetite and satiety that your body sends you, you can support your overall health and weight maintenance.

10. One potential strategy is to set aside a portion of each week for meal preparation in batches. Carry out ingredient preparation in bulk, including the preparation of cereals, slicing vegetables, and marinating proteins. During hectic weekdays, this can help save time and simplify the process of preparing nutritious meals.

11. Adopt a Moderate Approach and Flexibility: Maintain a flexible meal plan to accommodate dietary preferences, social obligations, or appetites. Moderate consumption of a diversity of foods is vital for developing a healthy relationship with food.

12. It is advisable to consult a registered dietitian or healthcare professional to obtain personalized guidance. They possess the ability to offer customized suggestions according to an individual's health requirements and assist in navigating dietary decisions that are consistent with the management of uterine fibroids.

By applying these suggestions for meal preparation and planning, individuals can establish a nourishing and well-balanced eating regimen that promotes overall health and potentially aids in the management of symptoms associated with uterine fibroids. Moreover, embracing a constructive perspective regarding dietary and lifestyle decisions enhances one's holistic state of being.

CHAPTER FIVE

The Utilization Of Dietary Supplements And Herbs

Fibroids of the uterus, which are benign protuberances, impact millions of women globally. Although medical treatments for fibroids are available, dietary modifications, with an emphasis on supplementation with botanicals, are an emerging method of managing this condition. Natural elements have the potential to alleviate symptoms and promote overall uterine health.

Herbal supplements and herbs are essential in mitigating the hormonal disruptions that are linked to uterine fibroids. The ability of Vitex, also known as chasteberry, to regulate hormonal fluctuations is well-known.

In addition, red clover and ginger herbal teas have the potential to reduce inflammation and mitigate discomfort. Vitamin D and omega-3 fatty acids are essential for managing fibroids as they promote a healthy hormonal balance and strengthen the immune system.

Incorporating these supplements and botanicals into one's daily regimen necessitates a deliberate procedure. It is imperative to seek guidance from a healthcare professional or a nutritionist to ascertain the optimal dosage and combination of botanicals and supplements that cater to one's specific requirements. Although these natural remedies exhibit potential, they ought to be regarded as supplementary to conventional medical interventions, thus constituting a comprehensive strategy for the management of uterine fibroid.

Changes In Lifestyle For Uterine Health

The development of a cookbook on uterine fibroids entails not only the careful selection of ingredients but also a more comprehensive dedication to adopting lifestyle modifications that promote uterine health. Adequate sleep, regular exercise, and stress management are all crucial components in the management of fibroids and the promotion of overall health.

Physical activity, specifically aerobic and yoga-based routines, has been shown to enhance blood circulation and mitigate inflammation. The implementation of stress reduction strategies, including deep breathing exercises and meditation, may have a positive impact on hormonal equilibrium, which is an essential component in the management of fibroids. Additionally crucial is sufficient sleep, as it facilitates the body's innate healing mechanisms.

Additionally, it is essential to maintain a healthy weight and prevent exposure to environmental pollutants. Specific chemical constituents present in household products and pesticides have the potential to disturb the hormonal equilibrium, thereby potentially worsening symptoms associated with fibroid. Adhering to a well-rounded diet that is abundant in whole cereals, fruits, and vegetables not only aids in weight control but also supplies vital nutrients that are indispensable for uterine health.

Adopting these lifestyle adjustments necessitates a comprehensive dedication to one's overall welfare. By incorporating these practices into their daily regimens, individuals have the potential to fortify the resilience of their bodies and mitigate the adverse effects that uterine fibroids may have on their lives.

Intentional Eating Methods

A transformative practice, mindful nutrition has the potential to have a substantial impact on the management of uterine fibroids. This strategy emphasizes making deliberate food selections, being fully present during meals, and paying attention to appetite and fullness indicators. A mindful dietary practice has the potential to enhance digestion, nutrient assimilation, and emotional well-being in individuals who are managing fibroids.

Savoring each morsel, thoroughly chewing food, and appreciating its flavors and textures constitute mindful dining. An improved relationship with food can be achieved through the practice of slowing down and tuning into the body's signals. This is especially crucial for individuals who have fibroids, as specific dietary decisions have the potential to impact hormone levels and inflammation.

A uterine fibroids cookbook that incorporates mindful eating practices should emphasize the following: portion control, selection of nutrient-dense foods, and identification of emotional triggers that may contribute to unhealthful eating behaviors. By cultivating a conscientious attitude towards food, people can enable themselves to make decisions that promote their holistic welfare and specifically tackle the obstacles presented by uterine fibroids.

Illustrative Meal Plans

To compile a cookbook on uterine fibroids, meal plans must be designed with an emphasis on ingredients recognized for their beneficial effects on uterine health. A meticulously organized meal regimen ought to incorporate an assortment of fruits, vegetables, whole cereals, and lean proteins while restricting the consumption of refined foods, caffeine, and alcohol.

A smoothie containing berries, kale, and flaxseeds could be offered for breakfast, providing a nutrient-dense beginning to the day.

For lunch, one might assemble a quinoa salad accompanied by vibrant vegetables and grilled chicken, thereby achieving a harmonious combination of protein and fiber. Salmon served alongside sautéed broccoli and sweet potatoes for supper is an excellent source of omega-3 fatty acids and vital nutrients.

Snacks, such as a fistful of almonds or Greek yogurt accompanied by fresh fruit, can be selected with intention. Proper hydration is of the utmost importance; water and medicinal infusions are favored options.

It is essential to tailor meal plans to the preferences and dietary restrictions of each individual. Seeking guidance from a healthcare professional or a nutritionist can be beneficial in customizing meal plans to suit particular requirements, guaranteeing that they are to individual preferences and the objective of effectively managing uterine fibroids.

Frequently Asked Questions

1. Is diet a standalone treatment for uterine fibroids?

A healthy diet may aid in symptom management, but it is improbable to eradicate fibroids. Dietary modifications ought to be regarded as a supplementary strategy in conjunction with medical interventions.

2. When can one expect to observe the effects of dietary modifications?

The duration required to observe outcomes differs among individuals. Alongside other lifestyle modifications, consistent adherence to a cookbook for uterine fibroids may result in the incremental alleviation of symptoms over the course of several months.

3. Should certain substances be avoided in the presence of uterine fibroids?

By limiting or eschewing caffeine, alcohol, processed foods, and red meat, some individuals may find relief. However, dietary recommendations ought to be tailored to the specific requirements of each individual.

4. Are supplements and botanicals capable of interfering with medications?

As they may interact with medications, it is imperative to seek the advice of a healthcare professional before incorporating botanicals and supplements into one's routine. The advice of a healthcare professional regarding safe and effective combinations is available.

5. Should weight reduction be incorporated into uterine fibroids management?

While it is advantageous for one's overall health to maintain a healthy weight, excessive weight reduction is not always necessary for the management of fibroids. It is advised to adopt a balanced approach to both diet and exercise.

In summary, a cookbook on uterine fibroids serves as a potent resource for those in search of a comprehensive strategy to effectively manage this condition. Proactive measures toward uterine wellness can be implemented by individuals through the utilization of botanicals, supplements, lifestyle modifications, mindful eating, and personalized meal plans.

Furthermore, by responding to frequently inquired inquiries, individuals can obtain valuable insights that will assist them in their endeavor to manage uterine fibroids via dietary selections. Collaboration between individuals and healthcare professionals is imperative to develop an all-encompassing and individualized approach to the effective management of uterine fibroids.

Conclusion

In summary, the Uterine Fibroids Cookbook functions as an invaluable resource that enables individuals to proactively manage uterine fibroids and regain authority over their health and overall well-being. Through the integration of culinary proficiency and nutritional expertise, this cookbook presents a holistic strategy to assist individuals coping with uterine fibroids. The recipes that have been provided are not only palatable but also thoughtfully designed to incorporate components that may offer potential advantages in the management of fibroid symptoms.

The significance of a balanced diet in fostering general health and attending to particular issues associated with uterine fibroids is underscored in this cookbook. Every recipe, ranging from nourishing juices to hearty meals, adheres to the tenets of a diet favorable to fibroid syndrome by utilizing ingredients recognized for their hormone-balancing and anti-inflammatory attributes.

The comprehensive methodology of the cookbook is augmented by the incorporation of enlightening segments concerning dietary protocols, lifestyle recommendations, and possible inducements.

In addition, the Uterine Fibroids Cookbook promotes a feeling of camaraderie and assistance, recognizing the difficulties that individuals encounter while attempting to manage their health condition. Through the promotion of nutritional awareness and the cultivation of a positive attitude toward food, the cookbook endeavors to enable readers to make educated decisions that impact their overall health. In essence, this gastronomic manual not only furnishes an anthology of delectable recipes but also functions as a companion in the wider endeavor to effectively manage uterine fibroids and advocate for a more salubrious, harmonious way of life.

THE END